MUSIC *AND* SONG, MOTHER *AND* LOVE

Other Books by Dr. John Diamond:

Your Body Doesn't Lie

Life Energy: Unlocking the Hidden Power of Your Emotions to Achieve Total Well-Being

Life-Energy Analysis: A Way to Cantillation

The Re-Mothering Experience: How to Totally Love

The Life Energy in Music (The Life Energy in Music, Volume I)

The Wellspring of Music (The Life Energy in Music, Volume II)

The Heart of Music (The Life Energy in Music, Volume III)

A Spiritual Basis of Holistic Therapy

The Collected Papers, Volumes I and II

Speech, Language and the Power of the Breath

A Book of Cantillatory Poems

The Healer: Heart and Hearth

The Healing Power of Blake: A Distillation

The Way of the Pulse: Drumming with Spirit

Life Enhancement Through Music

The Veneration of Life: Through the Disease to the Soul

Holism and Beyond: The Essence of Holistic Medicine

MUSIC *AND* SONG, MOTHER *AND* LOVE

John Diamond, M.D.

ENHANCEMENT BOOKS
Bloomingdale, Illinois

MUSIC *AND* **SONG, MOTHER** *AND* **LOVE**
Copyright 2001 by John Diamond, M.D.

All rights reserved.

No portion of this book may be reproduced in any form without the permission in writing from the publisher.

Cover photograph by John Diamond.

Published by: Enhancement Books
                  P.O. Box 544
                  Bloomingdale, IL 60108
                  Website: www.vitalhealth.net
                  E-mail: vitalhealth@compuserve.com

Printed in the United States of America
ISBN 1-890995-33-9

*To all the many Musicians
I have been privileged to know.*

*And to all the Mothers,
each a source of Numinosity.*

*And especially to my Songstress,
my very own.*

You want
to sing
with love
and I want
to help you.
That's why
we're together.

INTRODUCTION

You have here virtually all you need to be able to make music without stress, and with fun, joy – and love.

And, whether you are a musician or not, how to understand music in a new, deeper way: how to feel and know its heart, to get closer to its very core, to feel its therapeutic power.

I have written in this "poetic" form in order to heighten my, and your, creativity.

These thoughts are the distillation of my over forty years of professional experience with music: in mental hospitals, in general hospitals, in psychiatric, alternative and holistic practices.

And most of all with people, just people, who aspire to grow, to realize themselves, to be as loving as possible, through the agency of that most powerful of all the creative modalities.

I have worked with so many of them – from world famous professionals, to those yet to sing.

To all I gratefully dedicate this book.

Music is not
physical,
nor feeling.
It exists in another plane.

May these little sayings help to take you there.

MUSIC AND MOTHERING

The Mother of Songs, the mother of our whole seed. [1]

Throughout the ages music has been associated with mothering. The first sounds the baby hears are those of his mother – her breathing, her pulse and of course her voice transmitted to him through his watery environment. He is in a sea of pulsation, all generated by the mother.

In the outer world when he is on her belly and at her breast, he still hears her pulsations and especially her voice. There is no sound more loving, more comforting, more divine, than the sound of the special voice that the mother uses for her baby. It is pure love, "the eternal musical instrument of heaven and earth."[2] Out of it arises the basic and greatest of all songs, the lullaby. The whole essence of music, no matter how complex and sophisticated it may have become, is based on the sounds of the mother. And all the healing powers of music relate to the divinity of her love for her baby, and the wish to fully communicate this to him, to relieve every stress and discomfort and bathe him totally in the glory of mother love. He is held and cradled and rocked and nursed and bathed to the sound of the mother's divine peaceful harmony.

Thus you may not be surprised to learn that we have found that the music of female conductors tends

---

[1] From a song of the Kagaba Indians, Colombia.
[2] John Ruskin.

to have greater comforting and therapeutic powers than that of most male conductors. Music is part of the mother's world. It is the great therapy.

Music invokes the divine love of the mother. It is her breath, her pulse, her spirit.

———

MUSIC AND THE MOTHER'S LOVE

The essence of music is the lullaby, the inherent desire for the mother to sing her love.

Music comes as love from the mother, The Mother. And is gratefully reciprocated to her, to Her.

And it is the task of the enlightened musician to constantly remind us of the Origin of music, of The Mother and Her Lullaby.

Thus music can be a great Therapy, filling us with Spirit, with Love – the true and only Healer. And the more the music is a pure communication of love, the higher will be its life energy, its healing power.

That is the reason for its existence.

The more heartfelt the interest, the more fervent the desire, the higher will be the Life Energy, the love, in the music. And the more freely the music moves with the Pulse, the greater will be its power.

Every factor that inhibits the free and complete acceptance and transmission of the love decreases the life energy of the music and blunts its true purpose. Everything from negative thoughts, to incorrect body usage, to unfavorable environmental conditions.

Every one of these factors can be assessed and optimized to release the greatest glory in the music.

Every sound, every note, every timbre, every chord, every phrase, gesture and motif, all have specific effects in relationship to specific emotional and physical states.

The essence of Creativity is the bringing forth of these therapeutic sounds from the wellspring of the creative unconscious. This comes from the composer's desire for love and peace for himself and for us. His therapy and ours.

There is a deep and fervent desire within us all for growth and evolution. It is this that causes the composer to write, the performer to play, us to listen. And all to respond with outpourings of love and gratitude for Her Love.

And inside us all, albeit inhibited, is the fervent desire to make music, to give it. To actually reciprocate the mother's love.

All the factors that impede our evolution, all of them, can be overcome by Love.

In its ability to reaffirm the mother's love, lies the power of music.

> The holy ones
> are those who have found
> The Mother in their mothers.
>
> Thus can music sanctify us all.

———

To My Mother

Mother of my soul, dearest mother,
It is your birthday; I want to sing
Because my soul, bursting with love,
Young as it is, will never forget
The woman who brought me to life.

The years pass, the hours go round,
But time stands still when I'm at your side
Because of your enchanting caresses
And your loving glances, so rapturous,
That make my heart, impassioned, pound.

Every day I pray to God
To grant my parents life eternal,
Because the touch of your ardent lips
Upon my forehead is such a joy –
No other kiss could be its equal.[1]

---
[1] José Marti. "A Mi Madre." Translated from Spanish by Elizabeth Glick, 2001.

The lap of Comfort,
the hands of God,
the home of the Lullaby.

The whole world,
everyone,
is your mother –
as she was
in your beginning.

To be one again
with her
is to find Love, again,
at last.

And Music, too,
comes from her –
and is the easiest return.

Songs are born
in the womb,
inmost heart
of Her heart.

                                        Lullaby:
                                        soft,
                                        but intense,
                                        whole-hearted.

          She sings –
          I am loved.

There is
giving love,
– or not –
and there is
giving love
for the love.

The three levels
of energy
in music,
and life.

Songs –
because
words matter.

                                                  Make the
                                                words
                                                matter:
                                                sing
                                                the character.

                        Sinatra
                        loves the words.
                        He'd never scat.

Classical singing
is art –
and artifice:
not natural.

Imagine you are
the voice being sung,
the string being bowed.

Song
and dance:
the One.

Sing
when you move,
and move
when you sing:
equal parts
of the whole.

Songs
as golden
beams
from the heart.

Songs
as silver
voices
of night.

Every song
a perfect haiku
– and every
life.

Her Voice
over
the waters.

Lullaby
to love song:
life-history
of music.

                      Lips kiss
                      and sing –
                      eyes smile
                      and dance.

Every song
a perfect Buddha
– and every
singer.

The sweetest sound:
the lilt of love.

        Harmony
        is implicit
        in every song.

                What
                matters the pitch
                when the song
                is love?

Your singing
takes you
to Heaven
– not Caruso's.

                                        Sinatra's role?
                                        – to help us sing.

The organs
of singing:
throat
and heart.

                                        A bird
                                        can't help
                                        but sing:
                                        we
                                        have to choose.

Every problem
in your life
is there – right there –
in your singing.

And they all
resolve
with every
cantillating note.

The audience
is your mother,
so is the music
– and you.

The world a
perfect song,
always.

The song
flies up –
the heart
aspires.

Singing,
dancing –
and free!

"Ars gratia
Artis"
– Hollywood.
"Ars gratia
Amoris"
– Cantillation.

                        Go to
                        the concert
                        to be inspired
                        to sing it
                        yourself.

        A song from
        your seat
        worth
        two
        from the
        stage.

The voice
is you,
the instrument
you must marry
– and you know
what that means!

                    Your song
                    can spread
                    and spread.
                    Singing
                    is contagious.

          I am loved
          by a singer
          who sings!

The
song
seeks out
the
pain.

                                        Deep songs
                                        rise up
                                        higher.

Every song
a potential
Love Song.

                                        Go in,
                                        go in –
                                        become
                                        the Music!

Music
is the most
personal art,
for the audience
is midwife
to its birth.

Some songs
are personal
and close.
These are the
better ones.

Beautiful tone?
– Who cares!
Beautiful soul?
– Yes!

To sing
you don't need
a teacher –
just a mother.

Mother-to-baby talk:
lilt, and softness,
and intimacy,
with a quiet intensity,
and, of course, the love.

And that's how we
should sing.

Music with love,
spelled with an M
– like Mother.

Ask your husband
if he's hungry –
then your baby.
The difference
is music.

Look how
that mother
is holding her baby:
hold your song
just like that.

Song:
our Salvation.

                    Every song a pilgrimage
                    to the holy
                    blissful mater.

The last resistance
to liberation:
women conducting.

Female conductors
bring out more love.
The orchestra
needs a mother,
not a general.

To come into
the world
to your mother's song,
and for her
to leave it
to yours.

With a song
in my heart,
I'll never
walk alone.

Cantillation:
singing from
Belovedness.

The soft
gentle hands
of the mother
rounded
in gesture
of love.

Follow
the hands,
know
the song.

She made
our eyes
to close,
but not
our ears.

Our ears
reaching out
to her distant music.

The more songs
you know,
the more helpers
you can invoke.

The desire
to love
through music.

To find the love
of your mother,
replicate, as an adult,
her lullabies for her.

The bass a
pulsating
lullaby
cradling all
that happens
above.

Everything is mother:
the composer, the music, audience, the instrument,
your voice,
your muse, and you.

The only criterion
that matters!
Is it
a message of love?

Trusting the song
as you take it in,
as it fills you,
and rocks you
to sleep –
like a contented baby.
Then is music
the food of love.

                                           I put on the record
                                           and nestle into Her lap.

          Rocked
          and sung
          into sleep:
          Orpheus,
          Morpheus.

Love is music,
for music
is the voice
of the muse.

                              Every song
                              distorts
                              The Song
                              for
                              no one
                              hears Her
                              perfectly.

In tune
with the Voice
of the Mother.

                                        All the world
                                        is song and dance
                                        – that's Her
                                        design.

Music:
first-born
child
of Love.

                                        Croon,
                                        don't bellow,
                                        the baby
                                        will cry.

Sing –
and She
smiles
even more.

The song doesn't
matter:
only what
you
– and we –
become
through your singing.

In the children's ward,
isolated.
Through the glass
she waves good-bye,
hiding our tears.

I turn on the radio:
"You're the Only Star
in My Blue Heaven"
– and I'm comforted,
safe.

Spirit
in Her world,
substance in ours.
Music
the go-between.

Everything
singing,
when you listen.

Songs smile
– like mothers.

It's easier
to sing
than play
– no notes,
just words.

Gratitude
– from *gwere*,
song of praise.

A Song
unreturned
is love unrequited.

The Goddess Music,
daughter of
Mother Love.

                        Deep in every song:
                        an inherent loving Truth.

Music is an
emissary
from The Mother,
Love.

Intimate,
simple and pure:
the perfect
sonata –
a lullaby.

                              Pure, pure
                              lullabies –
                              that's all
                              the world needs.

        Annotate
        a lullaby?

                        A song
                        with love
                        for the lullaby.

As all music
comes from her,
it is the way
to her heart –
and therefore
your own.

                          Cantillation:
                          songs my Mother
                          taught me
                          going Home to her.

Enter the world
where music
is real.
Not notes,
not sound
– but Music.

That's where
you'll find
Love.

Her mother sang to her
in the womb,
in her lap, in the crib.
And she would smile,
and gurgle in return.
Then they sang together
in the kitchen.
And she would make up
little songs in bed
and send them up the hall
to Mommy.
Now she sings to the world,
her mother,
lovingly.

And when her mother lay dying,
she sang her into Heaven.

Her sound
enfolds me,
swaddled and safe.

                Music
                intimates
                the Way –
                and its
                acceptance.

Interface
of voice
and air,
of air and ear,
of heart and heart.

Instruments
complement singing
– but can
never replace.

Don't use
a walkman –
be a singman.

A smile inside
opens the throat.
Listen –
the voice
comes alive!

Everyone
can sing
– novices
even easier.

The voice:
very portable.

Marriage therapy?
Sing duets.

A love duet:
sing as the Mother
to each other.

Sing to
the God
that each of you
are.
That's marriage
therapy!

If you don't
want to sing,
something's
really wrong.
You'd better start
– right now!

                A hospital
                as temple
                of song.

                        Don't treat
                        his disease –
                        lift
                        his singing.

        Music
        frolics
        in the fields
        of love.

Rock the pillow
in your arms,
pretend it's
a baby:
hear your singing soften.

In your heart
is a song
yearning to be born.

Sing from your heart,
send the lullaby home.

Melody
lyric –
yin
yang.

                The marriage
                of music
                and words
                – no better
                than most.

A song's like
the Big Rock Candy
Mountain –
no one
can eat it all.

Treat
the singing,
and
thus
the singer.

As
in music,
so
in life.

    Woman
    is Song
    Eternal.

The pulse
of Music:
the rise and fall
of the breast.

    Your desire
    to sing
    comes
    from Her:
    She wants
    to hear you
    sing.

Creativity:
going down
to the Wellspring,
the Fountain of Love.

                                To find
                                the supra-mundane
                                in the mundane.
                                The real Music
                                in the sound.

There is
no must,
no beat –
just Pulse,
and Kindness,
and Love.

Every moment
I'm a new song.

Music's reality
another dimension,
beyond acoustics –
supra-mundane.

Each breath
all life
Now!
Each breath absolute
resolution.
Every breath a haiku.

                                          A song with love:
                                          notes of grace.

Your head
in her lap,
her song
in your heart.

The words
magnify
the music
of love.

The gift of speech,
the blessing of song.

Poems scan,
but lyrics sing!

Surrender to
Music,
heart
and soul.

Music exists
in another dimension,
beyond voice,
acoustics, chords.

There it flows,
pulsates and dances
– but these are mundane,
words.

Love descends
on invocation.

　

The muse's message
is always love,
but we
so often misprocess.

　

To find love
we must shift
to a higher plane
– and that's where
music dwells.

Under
the surface
of the song,
deeper,
much deeper –
that's where
you'll find
Her.

Music
best translates
the Muse's message
into this reality.

            To follow
            the song
            down
            to its
            source.

Music
takes you up
in Her arms
and transports you
to the Gates of Heaven.

Now, just sing
one note of Love
and you're through.

If
you can't
sing it,
you can't
play it
lovingly.

A life of lyricism
– and we are born
to sing.

Shiva dances,
the world sings.

Movement and
song –
essential
concommitants.

"You can sleep
anywhere,"
the old traveller
proclaimed.
"Just listen
to the music
of the engines."

Noise
becomes
Music,
when we
recognize
the Way.

Sing
not to be
heard,
but
for It
to be
known.

We have to know
we are loved
before we can love
ourselves, or others.
This is
the true role of art,
as it has always been.

Music
transports
the earth
to God.

Music
is a great
vehicle
for the expression
of love –
a Rolls Royce
Silver Sprite.

Sing
into
Silence.

Poems sit –
songs soar!!

Music:
Spirit
encircling the globe.

To find
God
on earth,
seek Music
in sound.

There is an inherent,
deep loving Truth
in every song
that when you approach It
puts you into the exalted state
of Belovedness.

The lowest part
of the human brain
is called the reptilian.
That's how lizards
think and move –
on the beat.
And dyslexics –
and everyone when stressed.

The cure?
To sing, dance,
live,
on the pulse.

Beat: lizard,
pulse: kangaroo.

Why make music?
Why sing?
Why the need,
the desire?

To express love,
grateful love.

Later,
we can do this
with just
our existence,
but the way
to that
is through music.

Every noun,
verb, and
preposition:
glittering jewels
in a necklace of song.

The melody
should lift
the pulse
of the poem –
never superimpose
its own.

Lyrics
are made
for singing –
and so are
we.

I sing
with the waves,
the wind
and the rain
– organum, sort of.

Don't try to see
how loud you can sing,
but how quietly –
with maximum intensity.

Go on –
sing off key!
You won't die!

To sing
in that way
which best invokes
the state of
Belovedness.

I am love,
I am Music,
I am Mother.

                        Lullabies
                        flying
                        everywhere!

She sings,
the dove
descends.

                        My wounds
                        bathed
                        in song.

Quietly sitting
after the music,
each alone
with the Mother.

All
the world
one Voice.

Sing
to be
true
to your
deepest
self.

She rocks
and sings,
and strokes.
He gurgles
and smiles.

                    Heaven sings!!

            Birds sing
            because
            their mothers
            fed them.

With a transcendental singer
you can hear the Muse at play.

　　　　　Music,
　　　　　messenger
　　　　　of Love.

Sing everywhere:
every place
a shower.

　　　　　　　Why is the Buddha
　　　　　　　close-mouthed?
　　　　　　　Has he sung already
　　　　　　　– or is it still to come?

If I could get
to the Heart
of a song,
I'd know
Everything.

Music is the string
through the labyrinth
to Love.

The world
doesn't need
singers,
but lovers
who sing.

Songs
dance
from
hearts
aflame.

Music
the greatest
healer
for it
brings us closest
to Her.

Your heartbeat
against hers –
that's syncopation!

                                                  The first
                                                  music:
                                                  mother sounds
                                                  through water.

From the
wellspring
deep inside
little ripples
break
the surface.
Each a song.

Silent prayer?
Yes –
if the body
is singing.

                    All
                    those silent
                    joggers!

          To reveal
          the pulse
          and then
          lift it
          higher:
          singing
          as cantillation.

The healing voice
rocks and rhymes,
alliterates,
lilting and loving,
like a lullaby,
with pictures of peace
and perfection.

                        The ferry boat
                        to the land of love
                        runs on music.

                        Hear the singing
                        over the waters.

            All that matters
            is love,
            and music
            is the easiest route.

We have
the power
to create
from love.

Radiate
the music
as love.

Selfless,
transcendent,
grateful love.

It's not
the music,
it's the Muse.

Every song, every night
must be a new expedition
to find the Muse.

However gifted
your father,
the first music
– the first love –
is always from
your mother.

Look at your audience.
There's your mother,
there's your Muse.

And She's smiling,
arms outstretched,
heart open.

Please sing to me,
my Darling.

Most of all,
Music can be
our salvation.
We just need
to learn how
to invoke It.

Mother love
starts with
the baby,
the Muse,
the goodness
inside.

So play for her,
and she'll be
rewarded –
and so will you.

Music can bring
God down
to us,
or, better,
lift us
up to Her.

The music starts,
She calls.
I follow Her voice
to Her inner chamber,
my heart,
my soul,
my womb.

Not
singing to find God,
but to realize
that we are.

Our singing never
is perfect,
always a little
off key,
but the Song
is always Perfect
– and each of us
is that Song.

The love that you
play with
is yours,
but the love
that you play
from
is Hers,
flying back home
as a song.

The origin of music
was in a sacred ritual.
Yes – mothering.

Instruments
are not called
musical
just because
they make it:
they themselves
<u>are</u> music,
our fingers
transporting their song
into the audible world.

For a man
to really
sing,
he must find
his softer self.

                        Sing
                        from your
                        deepest center.
                        Show the glory
                        of God.

        Sing!!
        Reveal your
        Godliness!

By "sing,"
I don't mean
only melody,
but every thought,
every movement,
every beat and breath –
the totality
of your every moment,
the music of your life.

I place my voice,
my ego,
my whole self,
at the service
of my Muse.
May She sing
through me.

                    I'm so blessed
                    to be working
                    with music –
                    all day
                    with the Muse,
                    the Mother.

I'm not trying
to teach you to sing,
I'm not a vocal pedagogue,
but to help you,
through music,
to be more creative
in everything.

Don't think of enlightenment
– or anything else –
when you sing.
Just feel
the deep, deep
pulsation
of purest love.

Singing opens
my eyes.
Suddenly,
everything is alive
– brightly vital,
vibrating
with Existence.

                              To sing Her song
                              so truly
                              that She smiles.

Yes,
Shinran was right.
It's not
how many times
I sing it,
but just once –
as truly as I can.

I open my eyes
after singing –
everything bright
and vital,
fully alive.
Me, too.

Singing
vivifies all –
even the sun.

Only the true musician
sings deep,
down to the Pulse.
Most are superficial,
many don't even
break the surface.

It's not the singing
that matters,
but living
as if you are –
fully, freely,
heart wide open,
soul to soul.

                              To always act
                              as if Truly singing.

Hear the singing
from the ferry boat
to the Pure Land.
Every pilgrim
a True Musician.

Music exists
in another world
where Love alone
is real.

When we sing and play
– and listen –
we can bring It down,
make it mundane,
or fly up
into Her realm.

To cantillate through Her,
you must believe
that Music as your mother,
truly, completely,
deeply, eternally,
loves you.

And to do this,
you need to enter
Her world,
suspending judgement,
accepting all and everything,
as She does.

To have Heaven
right now,
here, on earth,
enter the world
of Music.
She is there,
waiting,
in your soul,
arms outstretched,
face wreathed in song.

The True Musician
must find
not just
his Perfection,
but everyone's.
Only then,
can he sing
heart to heart.

True Music is
the pure Muse message
sung in this world.

True Music
is not just singing,
but releasing
the Muse
into your heart,
then into the world.

Feel the love
of the Muse
in a song,
any song,
and send it back
to Her.

That's the start
of the end
of all suffering.

The muse is Creative Power,
the Muse is the Mother.
Every time I seek
the muse of a song,
the muse of a composer,
I get closer to my Muse,
my Mother.
I get closer to her Perfection,
and mine.

Heaven
is the world
of Music –
not music
in this world,
but us
in Hers.

When you feel loved
by the music,
it's the Muse
singing through the music.

It's not
listening to music,
sometime,
but being Music,
the Muse –
always.

                        Surrender
                        your self
                        to your
                        Muse.

If I cause my Muse
to become manifest,
then She will call
to yours,
and She, too, will appear.

And they'll sing and dance
of Love,
and Mother,
and God.

What am I trying to do?
To examine and optimize,
all aspects of music,
at every level
of being.
Not just to make music,
but to find the Muse,
and release Her
into this world.

                    By Creativity
                    the Muse guides us
                    to Cantillation.

            Just to bring
            Muse music
            into the world,
            releasing Her
            to plant kisses,
            like a butterfly.

Musing,
prayer,
imagery, imagination,
music
– all creativity,
can take us
to the land of Love
– and then,
bring It
into ours.

Surrender
to your Muse.
Trust Her
to do the work,
and have faith
that She will.

The child at play
is all Muse,
but with little ego
to serve Her.

The musician
is little Muse,
and much ego,
serving itself.

The True Musician,
dedicating his ego
to Her,
becomes, once again,
all Muse.

The Muse
never sleeps,
She's always
sending out
Her message.

But the more
clearly,
lovingly,
we call,
the more
active,
excited,
She becomes.

The child
inside:
all Muse,
all music,
in water.

                Music,
                treated as silence,
                holy,
                doesn't frighten
                the Muse.

                              She is Song,
                              She is Dance,
                              She is Music,
                              and I enter into
                              Her Perfect
                              Silence.

The Muse,
fleeing the ego,
burrows subterranean.

Music
entices Her out.

Prayer is
True Music,
aspiring for union
with the Muse.

The True Musician
reveals the Muse
through the song
of his everyday life.

The true musician
most surrenders
to the Muse.

The true musician
aspires
to be True
through Music.

True Music
is so much more
than singing.

It is the Love
of the Muse,
the Mother within,
revealed
by any means
– even stillness,
silence.

> True Music
> is the Muse
> released
> into the world
> by any means
> – especially
> stillness
> and silence.

The more I treat
my music as silence,
the Truer it becomes.

> True Music
> seems to be
> the easiest way,
> but stillness,
> silence,
> may well be
> supreme.

I teach
not music
but life,
using music
as the first
metaphor.

                                        Death
                                        is when
                                        your last song
                                        dies away.

Music,
for the true listener
– and all art –
has no meaning,
no message,
no emotion.
Nor any purpose
but to take us
to the Land of Love.

Not just
to help you
with music,
but through music
to Perfection.

To enter
the world of Music,
suspend all judgement:
no good or bad,
no right or wrong.
In Her realm
everything Is!

Each poem,
each song,
a spiritual being,
its holiness praying
for release.

Each poem,
every song,
a spiritual being
yearning
for release.

Caress
and kiss it,
just so,
and it comes
into life.

Am I singing this
to really help other sufferers?
Do I feel filled
with the Spirit?
Am I inspired?
Am I enthused to help?
Am I aspiring to find
their Spiritual Being,
and to help them
to find It too?

Music
is the Middlest Way.
It is median,
mean, and mode.

Music,
like Spirit,
is everywhere,
is everything.

May I now,
right now;
sing with such faith,
with such love,
with such knowledge of Belovedness,
that I will go to the heart of the Muse.
I may then find perfection,
heaven on earth.
And may I then
be an example,
an inspiration for others,
that I may strengthen their faith
in their Perfection.

In the womb, on the breast, and now,
the whole world is mother.
And how you feel about her
– how loved you feel by her –
determines your attitude to everything
in life – including music.

The task of life is to feel,
perpetually, constantly,
loved by her, your goddess, your muse.
And the way to achieve this
state of blessedness is through music –
when played and sung in acknowledgement
of, and gratitude for, her love.

Every song a gift of love for the love.

ENVOI

*W*ell, I've tried with these aphorisms to pass on to you what I have learned from my years of working with music, and musicians, and musicians-to-be.

If you are a musician already, I hope you can now play more freely, transcendentally. And if you've never played or really sung, may you now be encouraged to – for music is life itself!

As you have seen, we've covered many topics, but the basics are few:

> Music comes from your mother.
> She is your muse.
> She loves you, and always has.

Even her imperfections are a part, an essential part, of her own Perfection. As she is Perfect, so are you – and everything you do, especially your music. Now sing to your audience, real or imagined, of her Perfection, and yours, and theirs.

Feel her love, feel your gratitude – sing your song of love.

One song
– just one –
with pure, pure
love
will resonate
all your days.

Open your heart
– let the lullaby
fly home.

Dr. John Diamond

Dr. John Diamond, M.D., D.P.M., F.R.A.N.Z.C.P., M.R.C.Psych., F.I.A.P.M., D.I.B.A.K., specialized in psychiatry and then in holistic medicine, holding numerous senior clinical and university teaching appointments. He is a Fellow of the Royal Australian and New Zealand College of Psychiatry, a Foundation Member of the Royal College of Psychiatrists and a Fellow and past President of the International Academy of Preventive Medicine.

One of Dr. Diamond's most consuming interests over his forty years of research and clinical practice has been the relationship between the Arts and health. As the Founder of the Institute for Music and Health, Dr. Diamond has investigated, researched and refined many factors in the musician and his instruments in an attempt to maximize music's therapeutic power. Many of the problems of life may be overcome, each in its own way, by our Highest Creativity – making the best choice in every situation for life, joy and health. Of all the therapeutic modalities, the creative Arts, especially music, can most actuate the will to be well.

A healer, author, photographer, poet, composer and musician, he has taught countless musicians and artists, and his knowledge extends to all genres of music. As a Holistic Consultant, Dr. Diamond continues to use music – as the great therapeutic modality – to achieve overall life enhancement.

For more information, please contact:

The Diamond Center
PO Box 381
South Salem, NY 10590 USA
(914) 533-2158

mail@diamondcenter.net
www.diamondcenter.net